# Weekly Meal Plan

|  | Breakfast | Lunch | Dinner | Snack |
|---|---|---|---|---|
| Mon |  |  |  |  |
| Tue |  |  |  |  |
| Wed |  |  |  |  |
| Thu |  |  |  |  |
| Fri |  |  |  |  |
| Sat |  |  |  |  |
| Sun |  |  |  |  |

# Grocery List

| PRODUCE | MEATS | BREAD/CEREAL |
|---|---|---|
| | | |

| DAIRY | BANKING / SPICY | CANNED GOODS |
|---|---|---|
| | | |

| FROZEN FOODS | CONDIMENTS | OTHER |
|---|---|---|
| | | |

# Weekly Meal Planner

Week of........./.........

|  | Breakfast | Lunch | Dinner | Snack |
|---|---|---|---|---|
| Mon |  |  |  |  |
| Tue |  |  |  |  |
| Wed |  |  |  |  |
| Thu |  |  |  |  |
| Fri |  |  |  |  |
| Sat |  |  |  |  |
| Sun |  |  |  |  |

# Grocery list

| PRODUCE | MEATS | BREAD/CEREAL |
|---|---|---|
| | | |

| DAIRY | BANKING / SPICY | CANNED GOODS |
|---|---|---|
| | | |

| FROZEN FOODS | CONDIMENTS | OTHER |
|---|---|---|
| | | |

# Weekly Meal Planner

Week of........../..........

|  | Breakfast | Lunch | Dinner | Snack |
|---|---|---|---|---|
| Mon | | | | |
| Tue | | | | |
| Wed | | | | |
| Thu | | | | |
| Fri | | | | |
| Sat | | | | |
| Sun | | | | |

# Grocery List

| PRODUCE | MEATS | BREAD/CEREAL |
|---|---|---|
| | | |

| DAIRY | BANKING / SPICY | CANNED GOODS |
|---|---|---|
| | | |

| FROZEN FOODS | CONDIMENTS | OTHER |
|---|---|---|
| | | |

# Weekly Meal Planner

Week of........./.........

|  | Breakfast | Lunch | Dinner | Snack |
|---|---|---|---|---|
| Mon |  |  |  |  |
| Tue |  |  |  |  |
| Wed |  |  |  |  |
| Thu |  |  |  |  |
| Fri |  |  |  |  |
| Sat |  |  |  |  |
| Sun |  |  |  |  |

# Grocery List

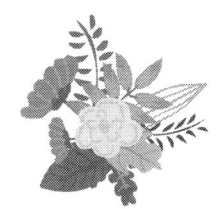

| PRODUCE | MEATS | BREAD/CEREAL |
|---|---|---|
| | | |

| DAIRY | BANKING / SPICY | CANNED GOODS |
|---|---|---|
| | | |

| FROZEN FOODS | CONDIMENTS | OTHER |
|---|---|---|
| | | |

# Weekly Meal Planner

Week of........./.........

|  | Breakfast | Lunch | Dinner | Snack |
|---|---|---|---|---|
| Mon |  |  |  |  |
| Tue |  |  |  |  |
| Wed |  |  |  |  |
| Thu |  |  |  |  |
| Fri |  |  |  |  |
| Sat |  |  |  |  |
| Sun |  |  |  |  |

# Grocery List

| PRODUCE | MEATS | BREAD/CEREAL |
|---------|-------|--------------|
|         |       |              |
|         |       |              |
|         |       |              |
|         |       |              |
|         |       |              |
|         |       |              |
|         |       |              |
| **DAIRY** | **BANKING / SPICY** | **CANNED GOODS** |
|         |       |              |
|         |       |              |
|         |       |              |
|         |       |              |
|         |       |              |
|         |       |              |
| **FROZEN FOODS** | **CONDIMENTS** | **OTHER** |
|         |       |              |
|         |       |              |
|         |       |              |
|         |       |              |
|         |       |              |
|         |       |              |

# Weekly Meal Planner

Week of........./.........

|  | Breakfast | Lunch | Dinner | Snack |
|---|---|---|---|---|
| Mon | | | | |
| Tue | | | | |
| Wed | | | | |
| Thu | | | | |
| Fri | | | | |
| Sat | | | | |
| Sun | | | | |

# Grocery List

| PRODUCE | MEATS | BREAD/CEREAL |
|---|---|---|
| | | |
| **DAIRY** | **BANKING / SPICY** | **CANNED GOODS** |
| | | |
| **FROZEN FOODS** | **CONDIMENTS** | **OTHER** |
| | | |

# Weekly Meal Planner

Week of........./.........

|  | Breakfast | Lunch | Dinner | Snack |
|---|---|---|---|---|
| Mon |  |  |  |  |
| Tue |  |  |  |  |
| Wed |  |  |  |  |
| Thu |  |  |  |  |
| Fri |  |  |  |  |
| Sat |  |  |  |  |
| Sun |  |  |  |  |

# Grocery List

| PRODUCE | MEATS | BREAD/CEREAL |
|---|---|---|
| | | |
| **DAIRY** | **BANKING / SPICY** | **CANNED GOODS** |
| | | |
| **FROZEN FOODS** | **CONDIMENTS** | **OTHER** |
| | | |

# Weekly Meal Planner

Week of........./.........

|  | Breakfast | Lunch | Dinner | Snack |
|---|---|---|---|---|
| Mon | | | | |
| Tue | | | | |
| Wed | | | | |
| Thu | | | | |
| Fri | | | | |
| Sat | | | | |
| Sun | | | | |

# Grocery List

| PRODUCE | MEATS | BREAD/CEREAL |
|---|---|---|
| | | |

| DAIRY | BANKING / SPICY | CANNED GOODS |
|---|---|---|
| | | |

| FROZEN FOODS | CONDIMENTS | OTHER |
|---|---|---|
| | | |

# Weekly Meal Planner

Week of........./.........

|  | Breakfast | Lunch | Dinner | Snack |
|---|---|---|---|---|
| Mon |  |  |  |  |
| Tue |  |  |  |  |
| Wed |  |  |  |  |
| Thu |  |  |  |  |
| Fri |  |  |  |  |
| Sat |  |  |  |  |
| Sun |  |  |  |  |

# Grocery List

| PRODUCE | MEATS | BREAD/CEREAL |
|---|---|---|
| | | |

| DAIRY | BANKING / SPICY | CANNED GOODS |
|---|---|---|
| | | |

| FROZEN FOODS | CONDIMENTS | OTHER |
|---|---|---|
| | | |

# Weekly Meal Planner

Week of........./.........

|  | Breakfast | Lunch | Dinner | Snack |
|---|---|---|---|---|
| Mon |  |  |  |  |
| Tue |  |  |  |  |
| Wed |  |  |  |  |
| Thu |  |  |  |  |
| Fri |  |  |  |  |
| Sat |  |  |  |  |
| Sun |  |  |  |  |

# Grocery List

| PRODUCE | MEATS | BREAD/CEREAL |
|---|---|---|
| | | |

| DAIRY | BAKING / SPICY | CANNED GOODS |
|---|---|---|
| | | |

| FROZEN FOODS | CONDIMENTS | OTHER |
|---|---|---|
| | | |

# Weekly Meal Planner

Week of........../..........

|  | Breakfast | Lunch | Dinner | Snack |
|---|---|---|---|---|
| Mon |  |  |  |  |
| Tue |  |  |  |  |
| Wed |  |  |  |  |
| Thu |  |  |  |  |
| Fri |  |  |  |  |
| Sat |  |  |  |  |
| Sun |  |  |  |  |

# Grocery List

| PRODUCE | MEATS | BREAD/CEREAL |
|---|---|---|
| | | |

| DAIRY | BANKING / SPICY | CANNED GOODS |
|---|---|---|
| | | |

| FROZEN FOODS | CONDIMENTS | OTHER |
|---|---|---|
| | | |

# Weekly Meal Planner

Week of........./.........

|  | Breakfast | Lunch | Dinner | Snack |
|---|---|---|---|---|
| Mon | | | | |
| Tue | | | | |
| Wed | | | | |
| Thu | | | | |
| Fri | | | | |
| Sat | | | | |
| Sun | | | | |

# Grocery List

| PRODUCE | MEATS | BREAD/CEREAL |
|---|---|---|
| | | |
| **DAIRY** | **BANKING / SPICY** | **CANNED GOODS** |
| | | |
| **FROZEN FOODS** | **CONDIMENTS** | **OTHER** |

# Weekly Meal Planner

Week of........./.........

|  | Breakfast | Lunch | Dinner | Snack |
|---|---|---|---|---|
| Mon | | | | |
| Tue | | | | |
| Wed | | | | |
| Thu | | | | |
| Fri | | | | |
| Sat | | | | |
| Sun | | | | |

# Grocery List

| PRODUCE | MEATS | BREAD/CEREAL |
|---|---|---|
| | | |

| DAIRY | BANKING / SPICY | CANNED GOODS |
|---|---|---|
| | | |

| FROZEN FOODS | CONDIMENTS | OTHER |
|---|---|---|
| | | |

# Weekly Meal Planner

Week of........./.........

|  | Breakfast | Lunch | Dinner | Snack |
|---|---|---|---|---|
| Mon |  |  |  |  |
| Tue |  |  |  |  |
| Wed |  |  |  |  |
| Thu |  |  |  |  |
| Fri |  |  |  |  |
| Sat |  |  |  |  |
| Sun |  |  |  |  |

# Grocery List

| PRODUCE | MEATS | BREAD/CEREAL |
|---|---|---|
| | | |
| | | |
| | | |
| | | |
| | | |
| | | |
| **DAIRY** | **BANKING / SPICY** | **CANNED GOODS** |
| | | |
| | | |
| | | |
| | | |
| | | |
| **FROZEN FOODS** | **CONDIMENTS** | **OTHER** |
| | | |
| | | |
| | | |
| | | |
| | | |

# Weekly Meal Planner

Week of........./.........

|  | Breakfast | Lunch | Dinner | Snack |
|---|---|---|---|---|
| Mon |  |  |  |  |
| Tue |  |  |  |  |
| Wed |  |  |  |  |
| Thu |  |  |  |  |
| Fri |  |  |  |  |
| Sat |  |  |  |  |
| Sun |  |  |  |  |

# Grocery List

| PRODUCE | MEATS | BREAD/CEREAL |
|---|---|---|
| | | |

| DAIRY | BANKING / SPICY | CANNED GOODS |
|---|---|---|
| | | |

| FROZEN FOODS | CONDIMENTS | OTHER |
|---|---|---|
| | | |

# Weekly Meal Planner

Week of........../..........

|  | Breakfast | Lunch | Dinner | Snack |
|---|---|---|---|---|
| Mon | | | | |
| Tue | | | | |
| Wed | | | | |
| Thu | | | | |
| Fri | | | | |
| Sat | | | | |
| Sun | | | | |

# Grocery List

| PRODUCE | MEATS | BREAD/CEREAL |
|---|---|---|
|  |  |  |
|  |  |  |
|  |  |  |

| DAIRY | BAKING / SPICY | CANNED GOODS |
|---|---|---|
|  |  |  |
|  |  |  |
|  |  |  |

| FROZEN FOODS | CONDIMENTS | OTHER |
|---|---|---|
|  |  |  |
|  |  |  |
|  |  |  |

# Weekly Meal Planner

Week of........./.........

|  | Breakfast | Lunch | Dinner | Snack |
|---|---|---|---|---|
| Mon | | | | |
| Tue | | | | |
| Wed | | | | |
| Thu | | | | |
| Fri | | | | |
| Sat | | | | |
| Sun | | | | |

# Grocery List

| PRODUCE | MEATS | BREAD/CEREAL |
|---------|-------|--------------|
|         |       |              |
|         |       |              |
|         |       |              |
|         |       |              |
|         |       |              |
|         |       |              |
| **DAIRY** | **BANKING / SPICY** | **CANNED GOODS** |
|         |       |              |
|         |       |              |
|         |       |              |
|         |       |              |
|         |       |              |
| **FROZEN FOODS** | **CONDIMENTS** | **OTHER** |
|         |       |              |
|         |       |              |
|         |       |              |
|         |       |              |
|         |       |              |

# Weekly Meal Planner

Week of........./.........

|  | Breakfast | Lunch | Dinner | Snack |
|---|---|---|---|---|
| Mon | | | | |
| Tue | | | | |
| Wed | | | | |
| Thu | | | | |
| Fri | | | | |
| Sat | | | | |
| Sun | | | | |

# Grocery List

| PRODUCE | MEATS | BREAD/CEREAL |
|---|---|---|
| | | |

| DAIRY | BANKING / SPICY | CANNED GOODS |
|---|---|---|
| | | |

| FROZEN FOODS | CONDIMENTS | OTHER |
|---|---|---|
| | | |

# Weekly Meal Planner

Week of........./.........

|  | Breakfast | Lunch | Dinner | Snack |
|---|---|---|---|---|
| Mon | | | | |
| Tue | | | | |
| Wed | | | | |
| Thu | | | | |
| Fri | | | | |
| Sat | | | | |
| Sun | | | | |

# Grocery List

| PRODUCE | MEATS | BREAD/CEREAL |
|---|---|---|
| | | |

| DAIRY | BANKING / SPICY | CANNED GOODS |
|---|---|---|
| | | |

| FROZEN FOODS | CONDIMENTS | OTHER |
|---|---|---|
| | | |

# Weekly Meal Planner

Week of........./.........

|  | Breakfast | Lunch | Dinner | Snack |
|---|---|---|---|---|
| Mon |  |  |  |  |
| Tue |  |  |  |  |
| Wed |  |  |  |  |
| Thu |  |  |  |  |
| Fri |  |  |  |  |
| Sat |  |  |  |  |
| Sun |  |  |  |  |

# Grocery list

| PRODUCE | MEATS | BREAD/CEREAL |
|---------|-------|--------------|
|         |       |              |
|         |       |              |
|         |       |              |
|         |       |              |
|         |       |              |
|         |       |              |
|         |       |              |
| **DAIRY** | **BANKING / SPICY** | **CANNED GOODS** |
|         |       |              |
|         |       |              |
|         |       |              |
|         |       |              |
|         |       |              |
| **FROZEN FOODS** | **CONDIMENTS** | **OTHER** |
|         |       |              |
|         |       |              |
|         |       |              |
|         |       |              |
|         |       |              |
|         |       |              |

# Weekly Meal Planner

Week of........./.........

|  | Breakfast | Lunch | Dinner | Snack |
|---|---|---|---|---|
| Mon | | | | |
| Tue | | | | |
| Wed | | | | |
| Thu | | | | |
| Fri | | | | |
| Sat | | | | |
| Sun | | | | |

# Grocery List

| PRODUCE | MEATS | BREAD/CEREAL |
|---|---|---|
| | | |

| DAIRY | BANKING / SPICY | CANNED GOODS |
|---|---|---|
| | | |

| FROZEN FOODS | CONDIMENTS | OTHER |
|---|---|---|
| | | |

# Weekly Meal Planner

Week of........./.........

|  | Breakfast | Lunch | Dinner | Snack |
|---|---|---|---|---|
| Mon | | | | |
| Tue | | | | |
| Wed | | | | |
| Thu | | | | |
| Fri | | | | |
| Sat | | | | |
| Sun | | | | |

# Grocery List

| PRODUCE | MEATS | BREAD/CEREAL |
|---|---|---|
| | | |
| | | |
| | | |
| | | |
| | | |
| | | |
| | | |
| **DAIRY** | **BANKING / SPICY** | **CANNED GOODS** |
| | | |
| | | |
| | | |
| | | |
| | | |
| | | |
| **FROZEN FOODS** | **CONDIMENTS** | **OTHER** |
| | | |
| | | |
| | | |
| | | |
| | | |
| | | |

# Weekly Meal Planner

Week of........./.........

|  | Breakfast | Lunch | Dinner | Snack |
|---|---|---|---|---|
| Mon | | | | |
| Tue | | | | |
| Wed | | | | |
| Thu | | | | |
| Fri | | | | |
| Sat | | | | |
| Sun | | | | |

# Grocery List

| PRODUCE | MEATS | BREAD/CEREAL |
|---|---|---|
| | | |

| DAIRY | BANKING / SPICY | CANNED GOODS |
|---|---|---|
| | | |

| FROZEN FOODS | CONDIMENTS | OTHER |
|---|---|---|
| | | |

# Weekly Meal Planner

Week of........./.........

|  | Breakfast | Lunch | Dinner | Snack |
|---|---|---|---|---|
| Mon |  |  |  |  |
| Tue |  |  |  |  |
| Wed |  |  |  |  |
| Thu |  |  |  |  |
| Fri |  |  |  |  |
| Sat |  |  |  |  |
| Sun |  |  |  |  |

# Grocery List

| PRODUCE | MEATS | BREAD/CEREAL |
|---|---|---|
| | | |

| DAIRY | BANKING / SPICY | CANNED GOODS |
|---|---|---|
| | | |

| FROZEN FOODS | CONDIMENTS | OTHER |
|---|---|---|
| | | |

# Weekly Meal Planner

Week of........../..........

|  | Breakfast | Lunch | Dinner | Snack |
|---|---|---|---|---|
| *Mon* |  |  |  |  |
| *Tue* |  |  |  |  |
| *Wed* |  |  |  |  |
| *Thu* |  |  |  |  |
| *Fri* |  |  |  |  |
| *Sat* |  |  |  |  |
| *Sun* |  |  |  |  |

# Grocery List

| PRODUCE | MEATS | BREAD/CEREAL |
|---|---|---|
| | | |

| DAIRY | BAKING / SPICY | CANNED GOODS |
|---|---|---|
| | | |

| FROZEN FOODS | CONDIMENTS | OTHER |
|---|---|---|
| | | |

# Weekly Meal Planner

Week of........../..........

|  | Breakfast | Lunch | Dinner | Snack |
|---|---|---|---|---|
| Mon | | | | |
| Tue | | | | |
| Wed | | | | |
| Thu | | | | |
| Fri | | | | |
| Sat | | | | |
| Sun | | | | |

# Grocery List

| PRODUCE | MEATS | BREAD/CEREAL |
|---|---|---|
| | | |

| DAIRY | BAKING / SPICY | CANNED GOODS |
|---|---|---|
| | | |

| FROZEN FOODS | CONDIMENTS | OTHER |
|---|---|---|
| | | |

# Weekly Meal Planner

Week of………/………

|  | Breakfast | Lunch | Dinner | Snack |
|---|---|---|---|---|
| Mon |  |  |  |  |
| Tue |  |  |  |  |
| Wed |  |  |  |  |
| Thu |  |  |  |  |
| Fri |  |  |  |  |
| Sat |  |  |  |  |
| Sun |  |  |  |  |

# Grocery List

| PRODUCE | MEATS | BREAD/CEREAL |
|---|---|---|
|  |  |  |

| DAIRY | BANKING / SPICY | CANNED GOODS |
|---|---|---|
|  |  |  |

| FROZEN FOODS | CONDIMENTS | OTHER |
|---|---|---|
|  |  |  |

# Weekly Meal Planner

Week of........./.........

|  | Breakfast | Lunch | Dinner | Snack |
|---|---|---|---|---|
| Mon |  |  |  |  |
| Tue |  |  |  |  |
| Wed |  |  |  |  |
| Thu |  |  |  |  |
| Fri |  |  |  |  |
| Sat |  |  |  |  |
| Sun |  |  |  |  |

# Grocery List

| PRODUCE | MEATS | BREAD/CEREAL |
|---|---|---|
| | | |

| DAIRY | BANKING / SPICY | CANNED GOODS |
|---|---|---|
| | | |

| FROZEN FOODS | CONDIMENTS | OTHER |
|---|---|---|
| | | |

# Weekly Meal Planner

Week of........./.........

|  | Breakfast | Lunch | Dinner | Snack |
|---|---|---|---|---|
| Mon | | | | |
| Tue | | | | |
| Wed | | | | |
| Thu | | | | |
| Fri | | | | |
| Sat | | | | |
| Sun | | | | |

# Grocery List

| PRODUCE | MEATS | BREAD/CEREAL |
|---|---|---|
| | | |

| DAIRY | BANKING / SPICY | CANNED GOODS |
|---|---|---|
| | | |

| FROZEN FOODS | CONDIMENTS | OTHER |
|---|---|---|
| | | |

# Weekly Meal Planner

Week of........../..........

|  | Breakfast | Lunch | Dinner | Snack |
|---|---|---|---|---|
| Mon |  |  |  |  |
| Tue |  |  |  |  |
| Wed |  |  |  |  |
| Thu |  |  |  |  |
| Fri |  |  |  |  |
| Sat |  |  |  |  |
| Sun |  |  |  |  |

# Grocery List

| PRODUCE | MEATS | BREAD/CEREAL |
|---|---|---|
| | | |

| DAIRY | BANKING / SPICY | CANNED GOODS |
|---|---|---|
| | | |

| FROZEN FOODS | CONDIMENTS | OTHER |
|---|---|---|
| | | |

# Weekly Meal Planner

Week of........../..........

|  | Breakfast | Lunch | Dinner | Snack |
|---|---|---|---|---|
| Mon | | | | |
| Tue | | | | |
| Wed | | | | |
| Thu | | | | |
| Fri | | | | |
| Sat | | | | |
| Sun | | | | |

# Grocery list

|  PRODUCE  |  MEATS  |  BREAD/CEREAL  |
|---|---|---|
|  DAIRY  |  BAKING / SPICY  |  CANNED GOODS  |
|  FROZEN FOODS  |  CONDIMENTS  |  OTHER  |

# Weekly Meal Planner

Week of........./.........

|  | Breakfast | Lunch | Dinner | Snack |
|---|---|---|---|---|
| Mon |  |  |  |  |
| Tue |  |  |  |  |
| Wed |  |  |  |  |
| Thu |  |  |  |  |
| Fri |  |  |  |  |
| Sat |  |  |  |  |
| Sun |  |  |  |  |

# Grocery List

| PRODUCE | MEATS | BREAD/CEREAL |
|---|---|---|
| | | |
| DAIRY | BANKING / SPICY | CANNED GOODS |
| | | |
| FROZEN FOODS | CONDIMENTS | OTHER |

# Weekly Meal Planner

Week of........./.........

|  | Breakfast | Lunch | Dinner | Snack |
|---|---|---|---|---|
| Mon |  |  |  |  |
| Tue |  |  |  |  |
| Wed |  |  |  |  |
| Thu |  |  |  |  |
| Fri |  |  |  |  |
| Sat |  |  |  |  |
| Sun |  |  |  |  |

# Grocery List

| PRODUCE | MEATS | BREAD/CEREAL |
|---|---|---|
| | | |

| DAIRY | BAKING / SPICY | CANNED GOODS |
|---|---|---|
| | | |

| FROZEN FOODS | CONDIMENTS | OTHER |
|---|---|---|
| | | |

# Weekly Meal Planner

Week of........./.........

|  | Breakfast | Lunch | Dinner | Snack |
|---|---|---|---|---|
| Mon | | | | |
| Tue | | | | |
| Wed | | | | |
| Thu | | | | |
| Fri | | | | |
| Sat | | | | |
| Sun | | | | |

# Grocery List

| PRODUCE | MEATS | BREAD/CEREAL |
|---------|-------|--------------|
|         |       |              |
|         |       |              |
|         |       |              |
|         |       |              |
|         |       |              |
|         |       |              |
|         |       |              |
| **DAIRY** | **BANKING / SPICY** | **CANNED GOODS** |
|         |       |              |
|         |       |              |
|         |       |              |
|         |       |              |
|         |       |              |
|         |       |              |
| **FROZEN FOODS** | **CONDIMENTS** | **OTHER** |
|         |       |              |
|         |       |              |
|         |       |              |
|         |       |              |
|         |       |              |

# Weekly Meal Planner

Week of........../..........

|  | Breakfast | Lunch | Dinner | Snack |
|---|---|---|---|---|
| Mon |  |  |  |  |
| Tue |  |  |  |  |
| Wed |  |  |  |  |
| Thu |  |  |  |  |
| Fri |  |  |  |  |
| Sat |  |  |  |  |
| Sun |  |  |  |  |

# Grocery list

| PRODUCE | MEATS | BREAD/CEREAL |
|---|---|---|
| | | |

| DAIRY | BANKING / SPICY | CANNED GOODS |
|---|---|---|
| | | |

| FROZEN FOODS | CONDIMENTS | OTHER |
|---|---|---|
| | | |

# Weekly Meal Planner

Week of........./.........

|  | Breakfast | Lunch | Dinner | Snack |
|---|---|---|---|---|
| Mon |  |  |  |  |
| Tue |  |  |  |  |
| Wed |  |  |  |  |
| Thu |  |  |  |  |
| Fri |  |  |  |  |
| Sat |  |  |  |  |
| Sun |  |  |  |  |

# Grocery List

| PRODUCE | MEATS | BREAD/CEREAL |
|---|---|---|
| | | |

| DAIRY | BAKING / SPICY | CANNED GOODS |
|---|---|---|
| | | |

| FROZEN FOODS | CONDIMENTS | OTHER |
|---|---|---|
| | | |

# Weekly Meal Planner

Week of........./.........

|  | Breakfast | Lunch | Dinner | Snack |
|---|---|---|---|---|
| Mon |  |  |  |  |
| Tue |  |  |  |  |
| Wed |  |  |  |  |
| Thu |  |  |  |  |
| Fri |  |  |  |  |
| Sat |  |  |  |  |
| Sun |  |  |  |  |

# Grocery List

| PRODUCE | MEATS | BREAD/CEREAL |
|---|---|---|
| | | |
| **DAIRY** | **BANKING / SPICY** | **CANNED GOODS** |
| | | |
| **FROZEN FOODS** | **CONDIMENTS** | **OTHER** |

# Weekly Meal Planner

Week of ........./.........

|  | Breakfast | Lunch | Dinner | Snack |
|---|---|---|---|---|
| Mon |  |  |  |  |
| Tue |  |  |  |  |
| Wed |  |  |  |  |
| Thu |  |  |  |  |
| Fri |  |  |  |  |
| Sat |  |  |  |  |
| Sun |  |  |  |  |

# Grocery List

| PRODUCE | MEATS | BREAD/CEREAL |
|---|---|---|
|  |  |  |

| DAIRY | BANKING / SPICY | CANNED GOODS |
|---|---|---|
|  |  |  |

| FROZEN FOODS | CONDIMENTS | OTHER |
|---|---|---|
|  |  |  |

# Weekly Meal Planner

Week of........./.........

|  | Breakfast | Lunch | Dinner | Snack |
|---|---|---|---|---|
| Mon |  |  |  |  |
| Tue |  |  |  |  |
| Wed |  |  |  |  |
| Thu |  |  |  |  |
| Fri |  |  |  |  |
| Sat |  |  |  |  |
| Sun |  |  |  |  |

# Grocery List

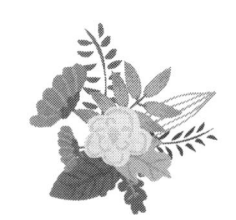

| PRODUCE | MEATS | BREAD/CEREAL |
|---|---|---|
| | | |

| DAIRY | BAKING / SPICY | CANNED GOODS |
|---|---|---|
| | | |

| FROZEN FOODS | CONDIMENTS | OTHER |
|---|---|---|
| | | |

# Weekly Meal Planner

Week of........./.........

|  | Breakfast | Lunch | Dinner | Snack |
|---|---|---|---|---|
| Mon |  |  |  |  |
| Tue |  |  |  |  |
| Wed |  |  |  |  |
| Thu |  |  |  |  |
| Fri |  |  |  |  |
| Sat |  |  |  |  |
| Sun |  |  |  |  |

# Grocery List

| PRODUCE | MEATS | BREAD/CEREAL |
|---|---|---|
| | | |
| **DAIRY** | **BANKING / SPICY** | **CANNED GOODS** |
| | | |
| **FROZEN FOODS** | **CONDIMENTS** | **OTHER** |

# Weekly Meal Planner

Week of........../..........

|     | Breakfast | Lunch | Dinner | Snack |
|-----|-----------|-------|--------|-------|
| Mon |           |       |        |       |
| Tue |           |       |        |       |
| Wed |           |       |        |       |
| Thu |           |       |        |       |
| Fri |           |       |        |       |
| Sat |           |       |        |       |
| Sun |           |       |        |       |

# Grocery List

| PRODUCE | MEATS | BREAD/CEREAL |
|---------|-------|--------------|
|         |       |              |
|         |       |              |
|         |       |              |
|         |       |              |
|         |       |              |
|         |       |              |

| DAIRY | BANKING / SPICY | CANNED GOODS |
|-------|-----------------|--------------|
|       |                 |              |
|       |                 |              |
|       |                 |              |
|       |                 |              |
|       |                 |              |
|       |                 |              |

| FROZEN FOODS | CONDIMENTS | OTHER |
|--------------|------------|-------|
|              |            |       |
|              |            |       |
|              |            |       |
|              |            |       |
|              |            |       |
|              |            |       |

# Weekly Meal Planner

Week of........./.........

|  | Breakfast | Lunch | Dinner | Snack |
|---|---|---|---|---|
| Mon |  |  |  |  |
| Tue |  |  |  |  |
| Wed |  |  |  |  |
| Thu |  |  |  |  |
| Fri |  |  |  |  |
| Sat |  |  |  |  |
| Sun |  |  |  |  |

# Grocery List

| PRODUCE | MEATS | BREAD/CEREAL |
|---|---|---|
| | | |

| DAIRY | BANKING / SPICY | CANNED GOODS |
|---|---|---|
| | | |

| FROZEN FOODS | CONDIMENTS | OTHER |
|---|---|---|
| | | |

# Weekly Meal Planner

Week of ........./.........

|  | Breakfast | Lunch | Dinner | Snack |
|---|---|---|---|---|
| Mon | | | | |
| Tue | | | | |
| Wed | | | | |
| Thu | | | | |
| Fri | | | | |
| Sat | | | | |
| Sun | | | | |

# Grocery List

| PRODUCE | MEATS | BREAD/CEREAL |
|---|---|---|
| | | |
| | | |
| | | |
| | | |
| | | |
| | | |
| **DAIRY** | **BANKING / SPICY** | **CANNED GOODS** |
| | | |
| | | |
| | | |
| | | |
| | | |
| **FROZEN FOODS** | **CONDIMENTS** | **OTHER** |
| | | |
| | | |
| | | |
| | | |
| | | |

# Weekly Meal Planner

Week of........./.........

|  | Breakfast | Lunch | Dinner | Snack |
|---|---|---|---|---|
| Mon |  |  |  |  |
| Tue |  |  |  |  |
| Wed |  |  |  |  |
| Thu |  |  |  |  |
| Fri |  |  |  |  |
| Sat |  |  |  |  |
| Sun |  |  |  |  |

# Grocery List

| PRODUCE | MEATS | BREAD/CEREAL |
|---|---|---|
| | | |
| | | |
| | | |
| | | |
| | | |
| | | |
| **DAIRY** | **BANKING / SPICY** | **CANNED GOODS** |
| | | |
| | | |
| | | |
| | | |
| | | |
| **FROZEN FOODS** | **CONDIMENTS** | **OTHER** |
| | | |
| | | |
| | | |
| | | |
| | | |
| | | |

# Weekly Meal Planner

Week of........./.........

|  | Breakfast | Lunch | Dinner | Snack |
|---|---|---|---|---|
| Mon |  |  |  |  |
| Tue |  |  |  |  |
| Wed |  |  |  |  |
| Thu |  |  |  |  |
| Fri |  |  |  |  |
| Sat |  |  |  |  |
| Sun |  |  |  |  |

# Grocery List

| PRODUCE | MEATS | BREAD/CEREAL |
|---|---|---|
| | | |

| DAIRY | BANKING / SPICY | CANNED GOODS |
|---|---|---|
| | | |

| FROZEN FOODS | CONDIMENTS | OTHER |
|---|---|---|
| | | |

# Weekly Meal Planner

Week of........./.........

|  | Breakfast | Lunch | Dinner | Snack |
|---|---|---|---|---|
| Mon |  |  |  |  |
| Tue |  |  |  |  |
| Wed |  |  |  |  |
| Thu |  |  |  |  |
| Fri |  |  |  |  |
| Sat |  |  |  |  |
| Sun |  |  |  |  |

# Grocery List

| PRODUCE | MEATS | BREAD/CEREAL |
|---|---|---|
| | | |

| DAIRY | BANKING / SPICY | CANNED GOODS |
|---|---|---|
| | | |

| FROZEN FOODS | CONDIMENTS | OTHER |
|---|---|---|
| | | |

# Weekly Meal Planner

Week of........./.........

|  | Breakfast | Lunch | Dinner | Snack |
|---|---|---|---|---|
| Mon |  |  |  |  |
| Tue |  |  |  |  |
| Wed |  |  |  |  |
| Thu |  |  |  |  |
| Fri |  |  |  |  |
| Sat |  |  |  |  |
| Sun |  |  |  |  |

# Grocery List

| PRODUCE | MEATS | BREAD/CEREAL |
|---|---|---|
| | | |

| DAIRY | BANKING / SPICY | CANNED GOODS |
|---|---|---|
| | | |

| FROZEN FOODS | CONDIMENTS | OTHER |
|---|---|---|
| | | |

# Weekly Meal Planner

Week of........./.........

|  | Breakfast | Lunch | Dinner | Snack |
|---|---|---|---|---|
| Mon |  |  |  |  |
| Tue |  |  |  |  |
| Wed |  |  |  |  |
| Thu |  |  |  |  |
| Fri |  |  |  |  |
| Sat |  |  |  |  |
| Sun |  |  |  |  |

# Grocery List

| PRODUCE | MEATS | BREAD/CEREAL |
|---|---|---|
| | | |

| DAIRY | BANKING / SPICY | CANNED GOODS |
|---|---|---|
| | | |

| FROZEN FOODS | CONDIMENTS | OTHER |
|---|---|---|
| | | |

# Weekly Meal Planner

Week of........./.........

|  | Breakfast | Lunch | Dinner | Snack |
|---|---|---|---|---|
| Mon | | | | |
| Tue | | | | |
| Wed | | | | |
| Thu | | | | |
| Fri | | | | |
| Sat | | | | |
| Sun | | | | |

# Grocery List

| PRODUCE | MEATS | BREAD/CEREAL |
|---|---|---|
| | | |

| DAIRY | BANKING / SPICY | CANNED GOODS |
|---|---|---|
| | | |

| FROZEN FOODS | CONDIMENTS | OTHER |
|---|---|---|
| | | |

# Weekly Meal Planner

Week of ………/………

|  | Breakfast | Lunch | Dinner | Snack |
|---|---|---|---|---|
| Mon |  |  |  |  |
| Tue |  |  |  |  |
| Wed |  |  |  |  |
| Thu |  |  |  |  |
| Fri |  |  |  |  |
| Sat |  |  |  |  |
| Sun |  |  |  |  |

# Grocery list

| PRODUCE | MEATS | BREAD/CEREAL |
|---|---|---|
| | | |

| DAIRY | BANKING / SPICY | CANNED GOODS |
|---|---|---|
| | | |

| FROZEN FOODS | CONDIMENTS | OTHER |
|---|---|---|
| | | |

# Weekly Meal Planner

Week of........./.........

|  | Breakfast | Lunch | Dinner | Snack |
|---|---|---|---|---|
| Mon |  |  |  |  |
| Tue |  |  |  |  |
| Wed |  |  |  |  |
| Thu |  |  |  |  |
| Fri |  |  |  |  |
| Sat |  |  |  |  |
| Sun |  |  |  |  |

# Grocery List

| PRODUCE | MEATS | BREAD/CEREAL |
|---|---|---|
| | | |
| DAIRY | BANKING / SPICY | CANNED GOODS |
| | | |
| FROZEN FOODS | CONDIMENTS | OTHER |

# Weekly Meal Planner

Week of........./.........

|  | Breakfast | Lunch | Dinner | Snack |
|---|---|---|---|---|
| Mon |  |  |  |  |
| Tue |  |  |  |  |
| Wed |  |  |  |  |
| Thu |  |  |  |  |
| Fri |  |  |  |  |
| Sat |  |  |  |  |
| Sun |  |  |  |  |

# Grocery List

| PRODUCE | MEATS | BREAD/CEREAL |
|---|---|---|
| | | |
| **DAIRY** | **BANKING / SPICY** | **CANNED GOODS** |
| | | |
| **FROZEN FOODS** | **CONDIMENTS** | **OTHER** |

# Weekly Meal Planner

Week of........./.........

|  | Breakfast | Lunch | Dinner | Snack |
|---|---|---|---|---|
| Mon |  |  |  |  |
| Tue |  |  |  |  |
| Wed |  |  |  |  |
| Thu |  |  |  |  |
| Fri |  |  |  |  |
| Sat |  |  |  |  |
| Sun |  |  |  |  |

# Grocery List

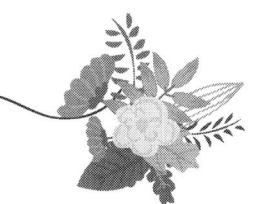

| PRODUCE | MEATS | BREAD/CEREAL |
|---|---|---|
| | | |

| DAIRY | BAKING / SPICY | CANNED GOODS |
|---|---|---|
| | | |

| FROZEN FOODS | CONDIMENTS | OTHER |
|---|---|---|
| | | |

# Weekly Meal Planner

Week of........./.........

|  | Breakfast | Lunch | Dinner | Snack |
|---|---|---|---|---|
| Mon |  |  |  |  |
| Tue |  |  |  |  |
| Wed |  |  |  |  |
| Thu |  |  |  |  |
| Fri |  |  |  |  |
| Sat |  |  |  |  |
| Sun |  |  |  |  |

# Grocery List

| PRODUCE | MEATS | BREAD/CEREAL |
|---|---|---|
| | | |

| DAIRY | BAKING / SPICY | CANNED GOODS |
|---|---|---|
| | | |

| FROZEN FOODS | CONDIMENTS | OTHER |
|---|---|---|
| | | |

# Weekly Meal Planner

Week of........./.........

|  | Breakfast | Lunch | Dinner | Snack |
|---|---|---|---|---|
| Mon | | | | |
| Tue | | | | |
| Wed | | | | |
| Thu | | | | |
| Fri | | | | |
| Sat | | | | |
| Sun | | | | |

# Grocery List

| PRODUCE | MEATS | BREAD/CEREAL |
|---|---|---|
| | | |

| DAIRY | BANKING / SPICY | CANNED GOODS |
|---|---|---|
| | | |

| FROZEN FOODS | CONDIMENTS | OTHER |
|---|---|---|
| | | |

# Weekly Meal Planner

Week of........./.........

|  | Breakfast | Lunch | Dinner | Snack |
|---|---|---|---|---|
| Mon |  |  |  |  |
| Tue |  |  |  |  |
| Wed |  |  |  |  |
| Thu |  |  |  |  |
| Fri |  |  |  |  |
| Sat |  |  |  |  |
| Sun |  |  |  |  |

# Grocery List

| PRODUCE | MEATS | BREAD/CEREAL |
|---------|-------|--------------|
|         |       |              |
|         |       |              |
|         |       |              |
|         |       |              |
|         |       |              |
|         |       |              |
|         |       |              |
| **DAIRY** | **BANKING / SPICY** | **CANNED GOODS** |
|         |       |              |
|         |       |              |
|         |       |              |
|         |       |              |
|         |       |              |
| **FROZEN FOODS** | **CONDIMENTS** | **OTHER** |
|         |       |              |
|         |       |              |
|         |       |              |
|         |       |              |
|         |       |              |

# Weekly Meal Planner

Week of........./.........

|  | Breakfast | Lunch | Dinner | Snack |
|---|---|---|---|---|
| Mon |  |  |  |  |
| Tue |  |  |  |  |
| Wed |  |  |  |  |
| Thu |  |  |  |  |
| Fri |  |  |  |  |
| Sat |  |  |  |  |
| Sun |  |  |  |  |

# Grocery List

| PRODUCE | MEATS | BREAD/CEREAL |
|---|---|---|
| | | |
| **DAIRY** | **BANKING / SPICY** | **CANNED GOODS** |
| | | |
| **FROZEN FOODS** | **CONDIMENTS** | **OTHER** |
| | | |

# Weekly Meal Planner

Week of........./.........

|  | Breakfast | Lunch | Dinner | Snack |
|---|---|---|---|---|
| Mon |  |  |  |  |
| Tue |  |  |  |  |
| Wed |  |  |  |  |
| Thu |  |  |  |  |
| Fri |  |  |  |  |
| Sat |  |  |  |  |
| Sun |  |  |  |  |

# Grocery List

| PRODUCE | MEATS | BREAD/CEREAL |
|---|---|---|
| | | |
| | | |
| | | |
| | | |
| | | |
| | | |
| **DAIRY** | **BANKING / SPICY** | **CANNED GOODS** |
| | | |
| | | |
| | | |
| | | |
| | | |
| **FROZEN FOODS** | **CONDIMENTS** | **OTHER** |
| | | |
| | | |
| | | |
| | | |
| | | |

# Weekly Meal Planner

Week of........./.........

|  | Breakfast | Lunch | Dinner | Snack |
|---|---|---|---|---|
| Mon |  |  |  |  |
| Tue |  |  |  |  |
| Wed |  |  |  |  |
| Thu |  |  |  |  |
| Fri |  |  |  |  |
| Sat |  |  |  |  |
| Sun |  |  |  |  |

# Grocery List

| PRODUCE | MEATS | BREAD/CEREAL |
|---|---|---|
| | | |

| DAIRY | BANKING / SPICY | CANNED GOODS |
|---|---|---|
| | | |

| FROZEN FOODS | CONDIMENTS | OTHER |
|---|---|---|
| | | |

# Weekly Meal Planner

Week of........./.........

|  | Breakfast | Lunch | Dinner | Snack |
|---|---|---|---|---|
| Mon | | | | |
| Tue | | | | |
| Wed | | | | |
| Thu | | | | |
| Fri | | | | |
| Sat | | | | |
| Sun | | | | |

# Grocery List

| PRODUCE | MEATS | BREAD/CEREAL |
|---|---|---|
| | | |
| DAIRY | BANKING / SPICY | CANNED GOODS |
| | | |
| FROZEN FOODS | CONDIMENTS | OTHER |

Made in the USA
Middletown, DE
30 March 2018